How to STOP Sugar Cravings

Discover How to Overcome Sugar Addiction and Stop Sugar Cravings

by Kevin Bryson

Table of Contents

Introduction 1

Chapter 1 – Causes of Sugar Addiction 7

Chapter 2 – Diseases Caused by Sugar Addiction 11

Chapter 3 – How to Eliminate Sugar from your Diet 19

Chapter 4 – How to Overcome Sugar Addiction 25

Chapter 5 – Improving Health by Overcoming Sugar Addiction 33

Conclusion 39

Other Recommended Resources 43

Introduction

You love sweets, and you think that nothing in this world could dissuade you from eating them. But what about the fact that sugar is also called "sweet poison"? And it can destroy your body, just like one of the zombies in the popular TV series "The Walking Dead"? Those horrible creatures feast on human internal organs as if they were succulent dishes. Ew, yes, but that's what accumulated sugar does to your internal organs, as well.

Excessive sugar obliterates your organs until nothing is left to perform their physiologic functions. In case you're one of the few, who haven't seen this TV series, then you may want to watch to see how this gory process takes place. But if you're already convinced of the importance of eliminating sugar in your diet, read on, and learn how you can overcome it.

When this craving for sweets happens regularly, you may have a sugar addiction. You love ice cream, chocolates and cakes, and you can't seem to feel full or satisfied after a meal until you've had your fill of these delectable desserts. Even your cup of coffee needs a generous amount of sugar for you to enjoy it. The majority of people actually do have a 'sweet tooth.' This is because the tongue recognizes the sweet taste first before other flavors, since the tip of your tongue is where the sweet taste buds are found.

Sugar is called 'sweet poison' due to the fact that large amounts of it in the body will cause several pathologic conditions, akin to the toxicity caused by poisons. The sad part is that sweets are not the only source of sugar in your diet. There are other sources of sugar that you may not even be aware of. One example is carbohydrates. Carbohydrates include things like rice, pasta, and potatoes, among many other food items. When these carbohydrates are metabolized by your liver, they are reduced to simple sugars called glucose.

Glucose (sugar) is the major source of energy in the body, but its level or concentration in the bloodstream should be within normal values so that serious pathologic conditions will not result. To put it simply, when the glucose level in your blood exceeds this normal level, and the body's physiologic system can't return it back to the normal level, this will result in a pathologic condition or disease called diabetes mellitus, which will be presented in Chapter 2.

Therefore, it's critical to eat only just enough sweets to provide you with the energy that you need for the day. Don't gorge yourself with unnecessary extra calories, which your body may not be able to burn or metabolize. If you're unable to burn those calories, they will add to the sugar content of your body and accumulate to eventually poison you. It's crucial that you learn what you're dealing with. Know your enemy and you'll triumph over it. Being aware of how much sugar you should consume is essential to your health.

Persons suffering from diabetes are not allowed to eat sweets because their pancreas cannot produce sufficient insulin, a hormone responsible in reducing the sugar content in the blood. The amount of sugar you can ingest will depend on your body's organ function, and your lifestyle. Since carbohydrates or sugar is the body's main source of energy, the more active you are, the more you'll be able to get rid of your excess sugar.

Next time you have that desire for another serving of your scrumptious dessert; don't give in to it, without fully considering all the damage it could do. That extra serving is detrimental to your health. That "just one more" slice of the sweet, yummy cake – especially if you tend to indulge frequently - is your sure ticket to acquiring type 2 diabetes mellitus. These pretty, sweet, seemingly harmless, foods are actually poisons-in-disguise that will eventually kill you.

For the sake of your own health, you need to eliminate your sugar cravings and overcome your addiction. Read on, and I'll help you discover how.

© **Copyright 2014 by LCPublifish LLC - All rights reserved.**

This document is geared towards providing exact and reliable information in regards to the topic and issue covered. The publication is sold with the idea that the publisher is not required to render accounting, officially permitted, or otherwise, qualified services. If advice is necessary, legal or professional, a practiced individual in the profession should be ordered.

- From a Declaration of Principles which was accepted and approved equally by a Committee of the American Bar Association and a Committee of Publishers and Associations.

In no way is it legal to reproduce, duplicate, or transmit any part of this document in either electronic means or in printed format. Recording of this publication is strictly prohibited and any storage of this document is not allowed unless with written permission from the publisher. All rights reserved.

The information provided herein is stated to be truthful and consistent, in that any liability, in terms of inattention or otherwise, by any usage or abuse of any policies, processes, or directions contained within is the solitary and utter responsibility of the recipient reader. Under no circumstances will any legal responsibility or blame be held against the publisher for any reparation, damages, or monetary loss due to the information herein, either directly or indirectly.

Respective authors own all copyrights not held by the publisher.

The information herein is offered for informational purposes solely, and is universal as so. The presentation of the information is without contract or any type of guarantee assurance.

The trademarks that are used are without any consent, and the publication of the trademark is without permission or backing by the trademark owner. All trademarks and brands within this book are for clarifying purposes only and are the owned by the owners themselves, not affiliated with this document.

Chapter 1 – Causes of Sugar Addiction

Before you learn how to eliminate sugar from your diet, you have to know first the possible causes of your addiction. Due to individual differences, people have various reasons why they are addicted to sugar. You have to find the reason of your own addiction to be able to get rid of it successfully. To cure any addiction, the root cause should be determined.

To find the reason of your sugar addiction, evaluate yourself honestly. Assess yourself using the following criteria, as points of references.

Sugar as a "comfort food"

Sweets are "comfort foods" to many people. They go into binge eating when they are depressed or anxious. What have you noticed about yourself? Do you also use sugar as a comfort food? Do you usually buy something sweet when you're down? Do you stuff your mouth with sweets after a break-up with someone you love? If any of these cases apply to you, then you're using sugar as a "comfort food."

Sugar as an Energizer

You've read somewhere that sugar can supply energy, so every time you need extra energy, you drink a copious amount of that sugar-sweetened beverage. Soon, even when you don't need that extra boost, you consume sweetened beverages because it has already turned into an addiction.

Sugar as a Palate Pleaser

Since the tip of the tongue is composed of the sweet taste buds, you may be one of the sugar addicts, who can't quite feel full if you don't have your dessert. Even your snacks may tend to be sugar-filled too. Do you usually have cake, cookies, chocolates, sweetened drinks, or ice cream as your favorite snack? Your affirmative answer indicates that this is the cause of your sugar addiction.

Sugar as carbohydrate

Sugar is used as a sweetener in preparing almost everything; coffee, cakes, ice cream, beverages, candies, and even entrees. Sugar improves the taste of food and drinks by its sweet flavor. In these types of food, you are aware of the presence of sugar because of their sweet flavor. However, sugar can be present in your food even if it doesn't taste sweet.

Carbohydrates are a good example. Carbohydrates, as previously mentioned, can come from rice, starch, potatoes, and pasta. Hence, you tend to ingest the sweet food not because of its sweet taste but because it may happen to be one of your favorite foods. Let's say spaghetti is your favorite food, and you eat it abundantly because you think that it has no sugar, since it's not sweet. In this instance, you become addicted to sugar without even knowing it; spaghetti is converted to sugar through the body's metabolism.

Take note of the reason why you might be a sugar addict, and keep this in mind as you continue reading, especially when we talk about overcoming your addiction through the methods presented in chapter 4.

Chapter 2 – Diseases Caused by Sugar Addiction

You're aware now that there are various diseases associated with increased sugar levels in your blood, which could eat you up, just like zombies. Your normal sugar level/concentration falls between the ranges 70 to 100 mg/dL for the reduction methods, and 60-110 mg/dL for the Orthotoluidine method.

The reference value or normal value for Fasting Blood Sugar (FBS) and related laboratory tests are method dependent, meaning, you should refer to the value given in the literature of the particular method performed on your blood specimen. An FBS value of more than or equal to 126 mg/dL, however, is the international value set for a possible diagnosis of diabetes mellitus.

If your body is not able to reduce your increased blood sugar back to its normal level, health problems will occur. As a sugar addict, you have to learn these scientific facts because knowledge will help in stopping your addiction. Here are health conditions and diseases related with uncontrolled sugar addiction:

Hyperglycemia

Your sugar addiction will definitely increase the blood sugar (blood glucose) in your body, and this increase in your blood sugar level (above the normal value) is termed hyperglycemia. The body has a built homeostatic ability to balance the substances in your bloodstream. This is only applicable, though, if your organs, endocrine, and nervous systems are functioning normally. Your blood sugar naturally increases after a meal but after about 2 hours, it should return to normal levels through your body's metabolism. The pancreas secretes insulin that helps reduce your blood sugar.

Diabetes Mellitus (DM)

When combined with other risk factors, such as obesity and family history, your continuous hyperglycemia could result in type 2 diabetes mellitus or acquired diabetes mellitus. Diabetes mellitus is caused by the insufficiency of insulin in the body. Insulin is a hormone produced by the pancreas that has the function of lowering the sugar level of the body when it's too high. Together with glucagon, another hormone secreted by your pancreas, they maintain the normal level of sugar in your blood.

Insufficiency of insulin is caused by pancreatectomy or the surgical removal of the pancreas due to a disease such as cancer or a tumor. It could also be caused by a dysfunction of the pancreas itself, or insulin resistance, which is the inability of the body to utilize insulin.

The US Centers for Disease Control and Prevention (CDC) has classified diabetes mellitus into 2 types:

- Type 1 DM – this usually occurs at an early age and is insulin dependent for treatment.

- Type 2 DM – this usually occurs at ages 40 and above and doesn't necessarily require insulin injection as treatment, but could use alternative drugs.

There are various differences between the two but for simplicity and for the purpose of this discussion, only basic info is presented to facilitate a basic understanding. Whatever type of DM you may have, your sugar addiction will exacerbate this condition.

Poor Wound Healing

Do you know that sugar serves as a nutrient for a variety of microorganisms? Microorganisms thrive on sugar, because your sweet blood feeds them. When you have a wound, it will fester and not heal. This is due to the rich sugar content of your blood that attracts more harmful microorganism to the wound site. Blood does not circulate properly into the peripheral capillaries either, preventing the entry of white blood cells (WBCs) into the wound. The WBCs are one of the factors responsible in helping heal your wound. So the lack of WBCs certainly slows down healing. This is also one of the symptoms of diabetes.

Polyuria

This condition is characterized by frequent urination. You may find yourself having to go to the john frequently. This is caused by the diuretic property of sugar. Sugar promotes water excretion or diuresis, so if sugar is present in large amounts, then you'll have the urge to urinate more often.

Polydipsia

This condition is characterized by excessive thirst. Think of your body as a vessel for drinking water in your home. When your family members drink more often, then you have to constantly fill the vessel to keep the supply going. This is what happens in polydipsia. Since you urinate more frequently than normal, you will have to drink more often too, to maintain sufficient water in your body. Your cells need hydration to perform their functions efficiently.

Polyphagia

This condition is characterized by excessive hunger. Some clinicians call it "hunger amidst plenty" because eating doesn't alleviate the condition. In most instances, eating will even worsen the condition. The reason for this is that the insufficiency of insulin in the body will prevent the proper metabolism and utilization of sugar in your system. You feel so hungry and weak even if you have just eaten because your body can't convert the sugar that you have eaten to energy.

The tendency is for you to eat more, thinking it will strengthen you, albeit, the opposite will occur. You'll grow weaker and weaker as you continue to eat. If you're a diabetic, your insufficient insulin will not be able to convert the accumulated sugar in your system into energy.

More complications of diabetes mellitus

Polyuria, polydipsia and polyphagia are called the classical triad because they occur commonly in diabetes mellitus.

Nevertheless, if your organs, central nervous system, and endocrine system are all functioning normally, then the hyperglycemia caused by your sugar addiction may be managed by your body properly through homeostasis. This means you'll won't necessarily get sick or experience these symptoms. As you grow older, though, your organs will also slow down, your metabolism slows down, and your hormones will not function like they used to. This is where serious health problems arise. Coupled with obesity, vices, lack of exercise, unhealthy lifestyle, and a family history of DM, you'll end up with acquired or type 2 diabetes mellitus.

Diabetes mellitus doesn't only encompass the conditions enumerated above but it also destroys all normal organ function. Your eyes, your liver, your heart, your kidneys, your lower extremity muscles and all the other physiologic and metabolic processes will be compromised. As a result, you'll increase your risk of cardiac diseases, genitourinary tract abnormalities, blindness and amputations of your lower extremities. Not to mention, you'll simply feel uncomfortable.

Unexplained weight loss or weight gain is another complication of DM. Usually the type 2 DM individuals are fat, while the type 1DM are thin.

In addition, diabetic ketoacidosis will result, when your body has to utilize fats as your source of energy. This happens when your system is unable to use sugar for energy. This abnormal usage will produce toxic substances called ketone bodies that will increase the acidity of your body.

Basic chemistry books state that the normal blood pH (acidity and alkalinity of blood) is 7.35 to 7.45, with an average of 7.4. In diabetic ketoacidosis, the blood pH becomes more acidic causing imbalance, and will eventually cause coma and death, if not managed appropriately.

According to the Centers for Disease Control and Prevention (CDC) of the US government, diabetes mellitus can, likewise, cause lower extremity amputations, and is *"the seventh leading cause of death in the United States."*

Chapter 3 – How to Eliminate Sugar from your Diet

Eliminating sugar in your diet is difficult if you don't recognize your sugar addiction, or especially if you're not willing to combat it. You'll need to become a smart food shopper, and read the labels of the food that you buy. Remember, not only sweet foods contain sugar but also carbohydrates. The primary purpose why you should eliminate sugar from your diet is to prevent you from getting sick from the side effects of accumulated sugar in your body. Here are healthy ways to remove sugar from diet.

Train yourself to reduce sugar intake

You need self-discipline to eliminate sugar from your diet. It's time to step up and claim responsibility for what you put in your mouth. Disciplining yourself will not be a ride in the park, but if you want to stay healthy and live a longer life, you must choose consciously to limit your sugar intake and, eventually, get rid of your sugar addiction. You can do it gradually by reducing the amount of sugar you place in your coffee or beverage daily. If you currently eat dessert after both lunch and dinner, then limit yourself to one dessert a day instead of two, and half the normal serving at that.

Use fruits in place of sugar

Fruits are excellent and healthy alternatives to sugar. Instead of drinking sweetened coffee during office breaks, you can have orange juice. Moreover, the caffeine content of coffee causes addiction, while fruit juice contains essential nutrients such as, vitamin C, calcium and other important minerals for your body's proper function. You could also choose carrot, apple or banana cake, in place of that creamy chocolate mousse cake. Make sure, though, that those fruit cakes are not full of sugar and milk.

Eating fruits as desserts is recommended by doctors because they are plenty sweet, yet healthier to eat. The sweetness of fruits comes from one of the simple sugars or monosaccharides called fructose. Glucose, fructose and galactose are the three most common dietary monosaccharides. Although fructose from fruits has almost the same effects as glucose, it's safer because it has a lower glycemic index than glucose. Glycemic index is a measure of how quickly your blood sugar rises after sugar or carbohydrate consumption. Fruits also have other healthy components such as fiber, vitamins, and essential nutrients, while sugars from sweets do not.

Reduce carbohydrate ingestion

Sugar when metabolized in the body becomes glucose. Likewise, the carbohydrates (rice, pasta, potatoes, bread) that you ingest are also converted to glucose through metabolism and the action of the hormone insulin. When you can't help but have a taste of that delicious birthday cake at your sister's party, make sure you reduce your carbohydrate intake that day so you won't be increasing, all the more, the levels of sugar (glucose) in your system. These increased levels will cause a multitude of diseases that could remain permanent.

Eat more vegetables

Like fruits, vegetables contain lots of fibers and important substances that aid the body in its physiologic functions. Eat at least 2-3 servings a day. Green, leafy vegetables provide natural anti-toxins and iron to the body, while yellow vegetables contain vitamin A. Vegetables also help the body get rid of excess unwanted acidic substances through their alkaline metabolism. When you learn to eat more vegetables, your desire for sweets will diminish because of the feeling of fullness that comes with eating vegetables.

Drink large amounts of water

Before, during, and after eating, drink lots of water so that you will quickly feel satiated. Don't be afraid to take in large amounts of this precious liquid. Your cells need water to grow and function properly. Your body is composed of around 70% water, hence, if you don't hydrate yourself sufficiently, think about those thirsty cells in your body drying up and dying. Water also aids in eliminating those harmful excess sugars, fats and toxic substances. A minimum of 8 glasses a day is required by your body. It's best to drink more water than the minimum requirement.

Exercise regularly

When your sugar addiction is tough to control, and you're still in the process of eliminating sugar from your diet, you can rely on exercise to burn the extra sugar in your blood. The purpose of eliminating sugar from your diet is to ensure that you remain healthy by maintaining your normal sugar levels. With exercise, you can do so, because regular exercise burns or metabolizes sugar in your body by converting it to energy.

Problems arise, however, when you have diabetes mellitus, wherein the body lacks insulin. Insulin insufficiency leads to hyperglycemia characteristic of a person with diabetes. In this case, exercising is not enough to manage the glucose level.

Chapter 4 – How to Overcome Sugar Addiction

Be positive. You can overcome sugar addiction if you really want to. Awareness of its detrimental effects to your health is enough rationale in doing so. Determination and self-discipline are crucial in overcoming your sugar addiction.

Based on your evaluation of the cause of your addiction in chapter one, you can now proceed to overcome it.

If you have used sugar as a "comfort food", you can now use alternative means to comfort yourself when feel depressed or anxious. Use these strategies as alternatives to sugar consumption:

- Listening to music – soft music can calm your nerves. Choose a genre that you feel most connected with, and listen to this in your room or someplace where you can relax undisturbed.

- Hanging out with friends – when you feel the urge to stuff yourself with those sweets because you're depressed or down, instead, go out and spend time with your friends. You can also open up to trusted friends about what's bothering you. This will provide an outlet for your depression.

- Taking a stroll in the park – having a breath of fresh air can ease your melancholia. Try it; it's free, healthy and refreshing.

- Developing a hobby – what's your passion? Develop a hobby from it and do away with the desire for sweets. You can get into photography, writing, swimming, dancing, or painting. There are countless hobbies you can select from. It's your choice.

- Spending time with family – family members are, usually, the closest people in one's life. If you have the support of your family, you can express your thoughts openly, while strengthening your bond. This is a superb way of doing away with sweets.

- Cultivating a positive attitude – you'll never resort to sugar as a comfort food, when you cultivate a positive outlook in life. You'll perceive each problem as an opportunity to grow and mature. You'll no longer spend sleepless nights worrying about almost everything in your life.

In cases where you use sugar as an energizer, a valid alternative is needed also. There are lots of energizing drinks that contain less or no sugar at all. So don't stick with the same one you've grown accustomed to. Instead, branch out, and read the labels of alternative energy boosters on the market or in your grocery store. Compare lots of them, and give the one with the least amount of sugar a try – you may have to drink it a few times before your taste buds have adjusted to liking it, but don't give up and go back to your old ways. Also, bananas are a good alternative for an energy boost because they contain sucrose and fructose, which will supply the energy you need, and simultaneously, provide healthy substances for your body, such as tryptophan, calcium, potassium, and vitamins.

If the cause of your sugar addiction is to please your palate, you can remedy this problem by using the following sweet alternatives:

- Fruits – as mentioned in the previous chapter, fruit is a good alternative for sugar because it contains fructose. Take note, nonetheless, that there are fruits with high glycemic index such as, mango, and those with low glycemic index such as, watermelon. In general, fruits are still healthier to eat than sugar.

- Raw honey – documented evidence from all over the world proved that raw honey has numerous health benefits. Aside from providing ample sweetness to food, it also helps cure many ailments such as sore throat, indigestion, and malnutrition. This is because of its antimicrobial properties, phytonutrients, antioxidants, enzymes, and carbohydrates. Make sure, however, that the honey you use is raw or unprocessed with no additives, so you can maximize its potential benefits.

- Molasses – You can use molasses if other alternatives (such as honey) are not available. This is still safer than refined sugar because it contains important minerals such as calcium and iron that are used by the body in biochemical processes namely, bone and red cell formation.

- Maple syrup – this syrup is a good and healthy substitute for sugar because it's sweeter and contains vitamins and antitoxins too. You can use this with cakes, beverages, and other foods that need sweetening.

- Stevia - this is an herb that is found widely in South America but is also commonly used in Japan. Recently, the US has labeled it, reportedly, as a dietary supplement. Stevia is sweeter than sugar but contains no calories; hence, it is ideal for use by diabetic patients because of its low glycemic index.

Avoid commercially prepared artificial sweeteners that contain aspartame and sucralose because intensive and extensive study is needed to establish their safety. Furthermore, according to reports, there were observed health problems, namely: migraines, seizures, toxicity and increased risks of cancer.

You can overcome your sugar addiction more successfully by being aware that there are foods that contain glucose, even if they are not sweet. Carbohydrates are metabolized to glucose so you should avoid them.

Avoid over-eating these foods because although they are not usually sweet, they contain sugar, or are metabolized to simple sugars, once they enter the body:

- Rice
- Pastas
- Grains
- Breads
- Dairy products
- Cereals
- Potatoes

- Yams
- Salad dressings
- Tomato sauce
- Coleslaw
- Any food made of starch

In cases where rice may be a staple food, unpolished rice should be your choice because, together with glucose, there are healthy components such as, Vitamin B, thiamine, minerals and a large amount of fiber. With regards to grains and bread, the whole grain and the whole wheat bread are preferred to prevent the occurrence of hyperglycemia.

By applying the aforementioned recommendations, you can overcome your sugar addiction and still be able to satiate your palate. And the amazing miracle is this: When you start to reduce your intake and consumption of sugar, your cravings will begin to disappear. Little by little, you will allow yourself less and less, and then as a natural reward, your body will want less and less. Eventually, you'll find yourself at a birthday party and the thought of that piece of cake will even seem repulsive or "too sweet" for you, and you'll turn it down without feeling deprived.

So one step at a time, implement some of these substitutions, reduced portions, and sugar limitations, until your new level of sugar intake begins to feel completely natural, and any additional sugar is undesired.

Chapter 5 – Improving your Health by Overcoming Sugar Addiction

Once you have decided to overcome your sugar addiction, you'll be reaping lots of benefits, including financial gains. You'll gain financially, in the sense that you'll be able to save more money on food, since you won't need to order an expensive dessert everywhere you go.

With numerous health conditions associated with sugar, eliminating sugar from your diet will have positive, significant results, to boot.

Your body organs are safeguarded

Because you no longer eat the "sweet poison", the circulating blood in your body is clean and pure. There are no toxicants coming from accumulated sugar from your diet. Your organs won't be overworked doing away with your excess sugar. Equally, your organs are protected from cell dysfunction and destruction due to hyperglycemia.

Your eyes are safe

You'll not worry anymore that you may go blind; close your eyes and imagine being in the dark for the rest of your life. Poor eyesight caused by diabetes is a sad occurrence; for the reason that it could have been easily prevented had the diabetic person knew beforehand the complications of his disease.

Your wounds will not harbor microorganisms

Your wounds will no longer be a nutrient hotbed for harmful microorganisms to breed and multiply. Your soldier-cells, the white blood cells, can now respond promptly to the site of your wounds to ensure that the healing process is started properly. You'll not be cowering in fear to have your ingrown toe nail be surgically removed, since you know it would heal in no time at all. Believe it or not, a festering wound of an ingrown toe nail from a bad pedicure is one of the reasons for leg amputation in diabetic patients. The wound nurtures pathologic bacteria that tend to spread to the entire body, if the leg is not amputated. You'll end up selecting amputation rather than death. Wouldn't you rather have chosen to eliminate or reduce sugar intake instead of amputation?

Your blood circulation improves

Think about a piped water system that effectively delivers water to your area. Because the water is not contaminated with sugar, there are no clogged waterways. Once there is sufficient distribution of water supply to all of the pipes, the people in that area will thrive. This is also true with blood circulation. Without the excess, syrupy sugar clogging or blocking your arteries or blood vessels, your circulation will improve and your cells will be nourished reliably.

Improved circulation initiates a number of health benefits:

- Facilitation of the transport of vital substances in the body. Blood acts as the "river" in which substances are brought from one place to another. If you're wondering how tissue wounds stop bleeding after sometime; it's because blood in the circulation brings platelets and clotting factors promptly to the site of the wound. These platelets and clotting factors are responsible in forming clots to plug areas where there is bleeding. The white blood cells are similarly transported readily to hasten tissue healing. Therapeutic drugs are also transported quickly to the tissues that need it.

- Elimination of unwanted toxic substances by the kidneys is enhanced. The faster your body removes these poisons from your system, the healthier you will be. Your kidneys are the main excretory organs in your body, and when there is proper circulation, there is also a reliable excretion of waste products.

- Cardiac function is ensured because your cardiac blood vessels can pump blood in and out of your heart without any problem, therefore, preventing the development of heart ailments.

- Respiratory function is enhanced due to the proper transport of oxygen through the arteries, and carbon dioxide through the veins. Improved circulation makes this biochemical process possible and efficient.

- Metabolic function of the liver is improved because there is no accumulation of sugar that would overload the process. The liver is the major metabolic organ of the body where foods, namely: carbohydrates, proteins and lipids are converted into their usable forms. The liver is also responsible in detoxifying the body of poisons or toxins by converting them into less toxic substances or water soluble forms, so that they can be excreted. Sugar or glucose is one of the substances metabolized by the liver through various biochemical processes. These are:

1. Glycolysis – is the breakdown of glucose to produce energy, when the body needs it.

2. Glycogenolysis – is the breakdown of stored glycogen back to glucose, when the body requires additional energy.

3. Gluconeogenesis – is the formation of glucose from non-carbohydrate sources such as, protein and fats, after stored glycogen has been depleted.

4. Glycogenesis – is the formation of glycogen from glucose, if glucose is not needed by the body.

All your organ-systems will be functioning normally; hence, you'll no longer experience the pain of polyuria, polydipsia, polyphagia, diabetic ketoacidosis, and all the other complications of hyperglycemia and diabetes mellitus.

The health benefits you derive from being free of your sugar addiction are tremendous. It's up to you now to take action.

Conclusion

Eliminating excess sugar in your diet and overcoming your addiction is possible. But you'll have to step up to the forefront and take charge of your health. Do you want to live your old age stuck to your bed or being physically disabled? Most probably, your answer will be "no"; thus, you should study all of this information carefully and make a positive commitment to do something about your sugar addiction. You have to be self-motivated and determined in eliminating sugar from your diet in order to succeed. It's only through your decisive action that your health will improve.

However, you also need to understand that getting rid of sugar doesn't mean starving yourself. Remember that your body cells also need sugar or glucose as a source of energy and nutrients. If you don't have sufficient sugar, this will result to serious diseases, as well. The sugar in the carbohydrate that's in your regular diet should be enough to provide the energy that your body requires on a daily, normal-activity basis. Hence, you can do away with your sweets.

When you need more energy, you can resort to the alternatives given in Chapter 4. Use the alternatives judiciously. Otherwise, do away with sugar, altogether. It's a sweet poison that will eventually destroy your body and cause health problems for you.

On the other hand, if you're a diabetic, then all the strategies presented here will work for you too, but on a stricter scale. Diabetes is a serious, life-long condition, hence, aside from following these methods and pointers, consult your Doctor or Clinician regularly for proper management and treatment.

During the process, you have to monitor your blood sugar to know whether you're progressing in your endeavor or not. A Fasting Blood Sugar (FBS) laboratory test, after an 8 to 12-hour fasting, can indicate if your sugar level is normal, or if you still have hyperglycemia. You'll know you're safe when you're able to get rid of excess sugar in your diet, and your blood sugar values are within normal limits.

Should you opt to ignore the warnings of sugar addiction now, you'll reap the dire consequences of your indifference later. While it's still early, curb your sugar addiction and stay healthy, because health is the ultimate wealth you possess.

Thank you for purchasing and reading this book, I truly hope it was helpful and informative, and that it will assist you in your journey to giving up Sugar. I applaud your decision to overcome your addiction, and live a long healthy life instead. Finally, if you enjoyed the book, I'd certainly appreciate it if you'd take a moment to leave a review for it on Amazon! Thanks again, and good luck!

Other Recommended Resources

Here are some additional resources I think you'll find helpful in your quest for a better body and healthier lifestyle.

1) **"Overweight No More: Ten Small Adjustments you can make Today for BIG Weight Loss and a Whole New You"**

    http://www.amazon.com/dp/B00KS4BBEW/

    http://amzn.to/1s5C79V

2) **"Exercise Motivation, Determination, and Discipline: How to Get into a Regular Exercise Routine, Stay Focused, and See Results Fast"**

    http://www.amazon.com/dp/B00LF9I7CI/

    http://amzn.to/1rfsIKe

3) **"WILLPOWER: How to Achieve your Goals by Making a Plan and Sticking to it with Self-Control, Discipline, and Ease"**

    http://www.amazon.com/dp/B00LH9NJZG/

    http://amzn.to/1m2rA7j

4) "Increase Metabolism: Start Losing Weight and Burning Body Fat Today with these 25 Effective and Simple Ways to Boost your Metabolism"

http://www.amazon.com/dp/B00KR0YOSC/

http://amzn.to/SwyM4e

5) "Self-Confidence: 25 Proven Ways to Boost your Self-Confidence to Overcome Anxiety, Fear, & Self-Doubt"

http://www.amazon.com/dp/B00LOWOQGC/

http://amzn.to/1kNdkQe

6) "Lose Weight Easily: How to Lose Weight (Without Weird Diets or Crazy Workout Regimens) for a Healthier Life"

http://www.amazon.com/dp/B00LQ99TMY/

http://amzn.to/1m2uOrn

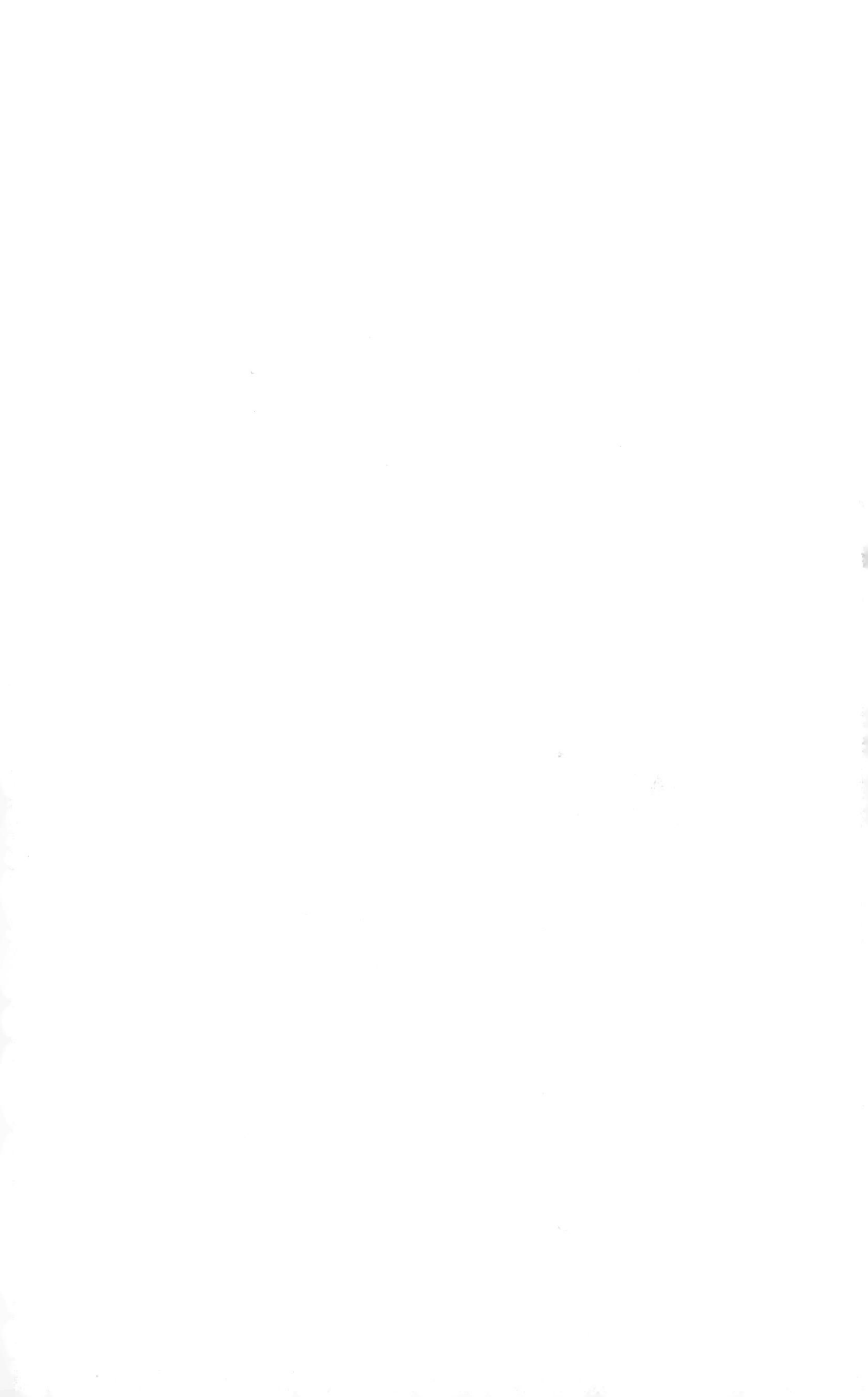

Made in the USA
San Bernardino, CA
05 July 2016